Brigitta's Mystical Garden Baby Bongo Book Series

Baby Bongo Learns To Swim

K.L. Hygaard

1

Baby Bongo Learns To Swim

"Brigitta's Mystical Garden
Baby Bongo Book Series"
– K. L. Hygaard

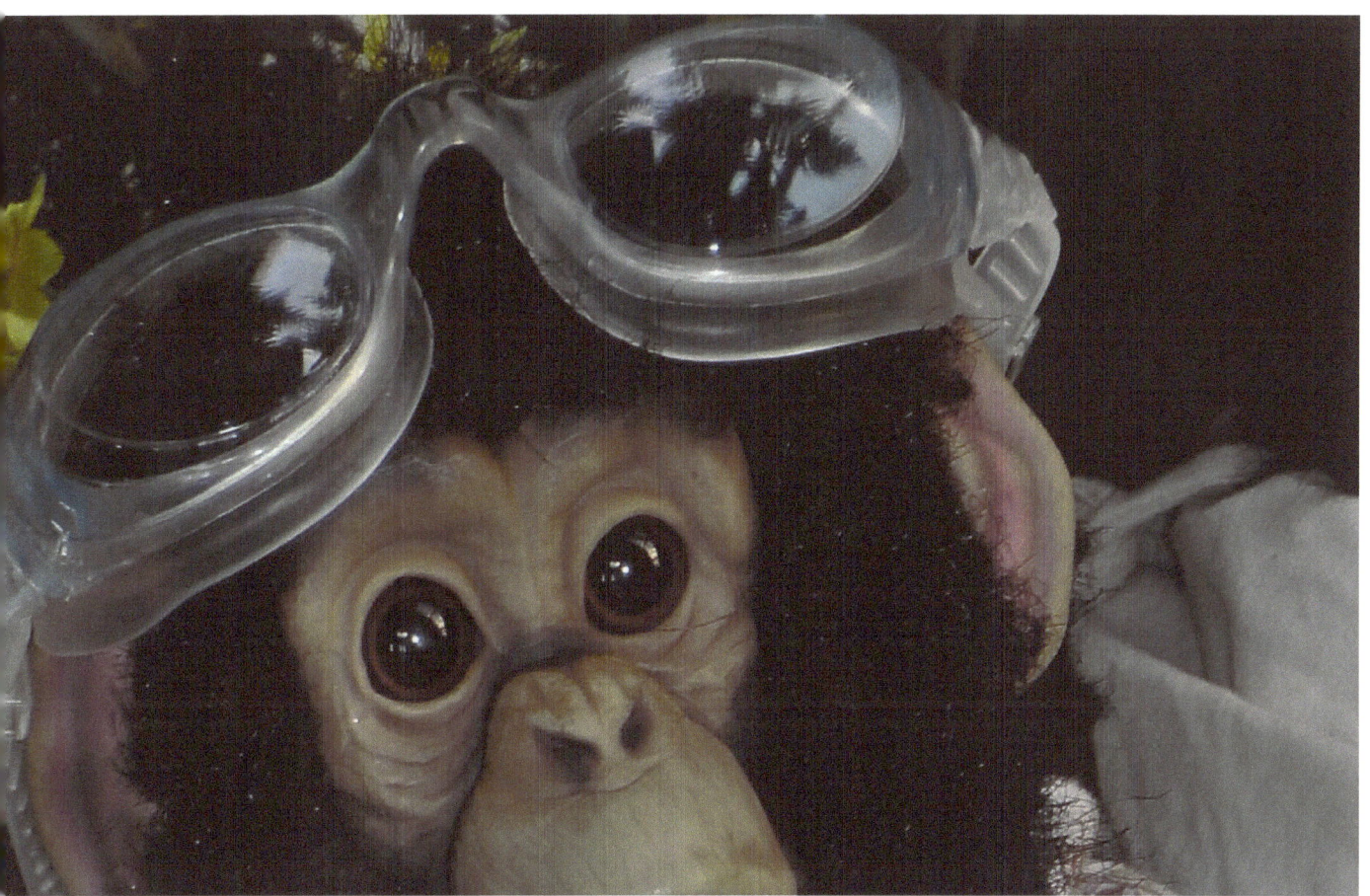

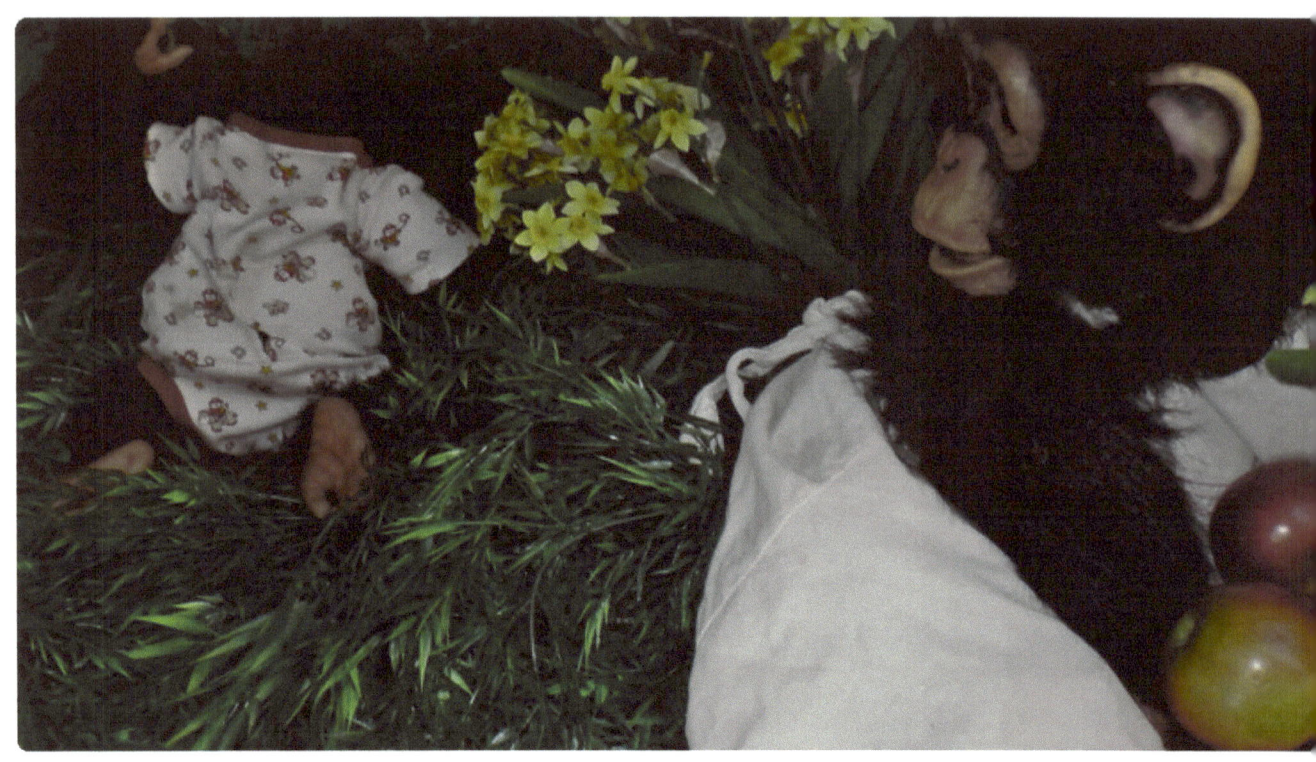

"Baby Bongo!" His Mommy sings out, "Time to get ready for your swimming lessons!" Baby Bongo gets very excited and starts bouncing up and down because he loves swimming and he gets ready right away!

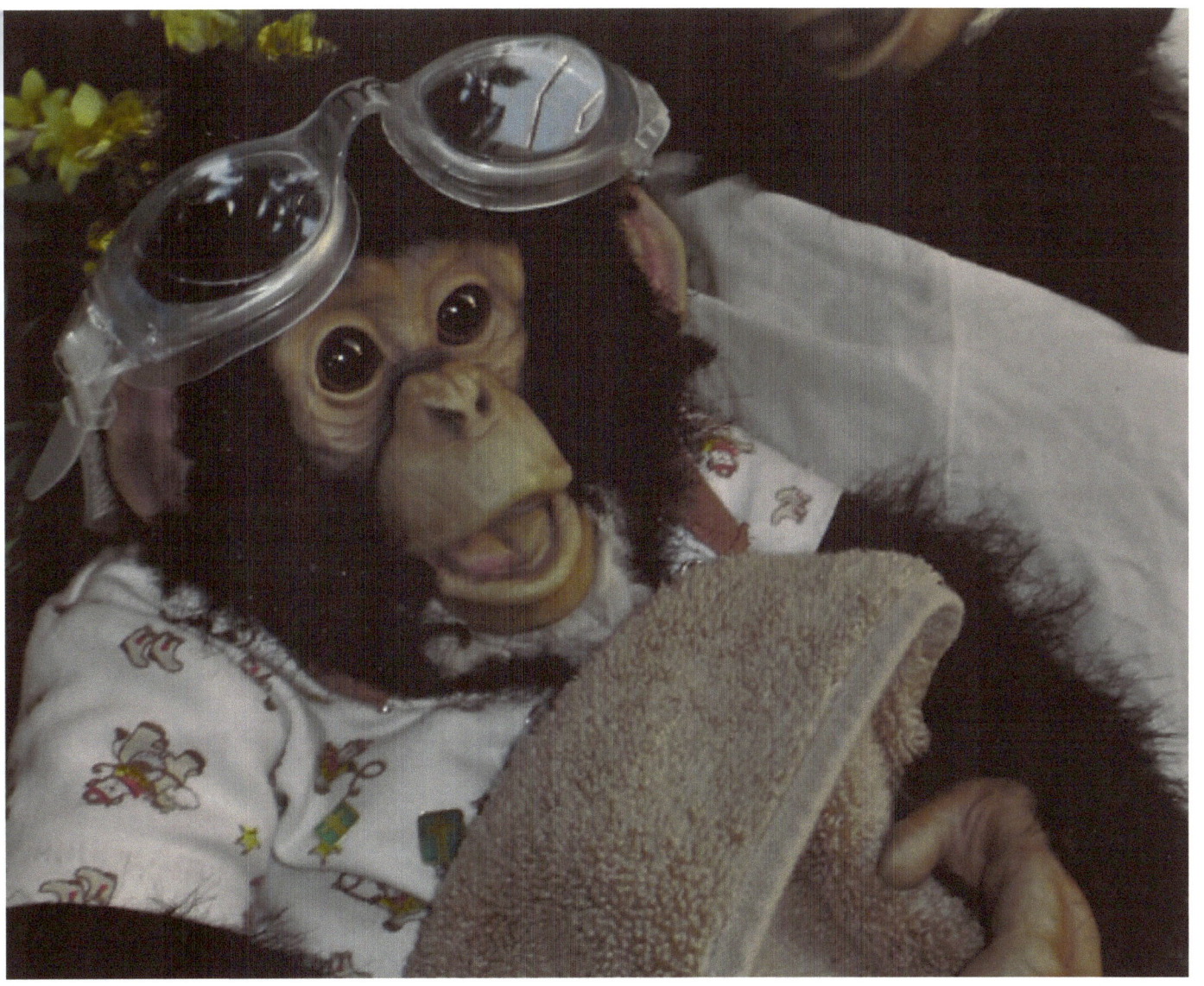

"Here are your goggles and towel, Baby Bongo!", says Mommy

as she smiles and her little chimp says "thank you"and quickly

climbs high in the treetops to see the water he will swim in today!

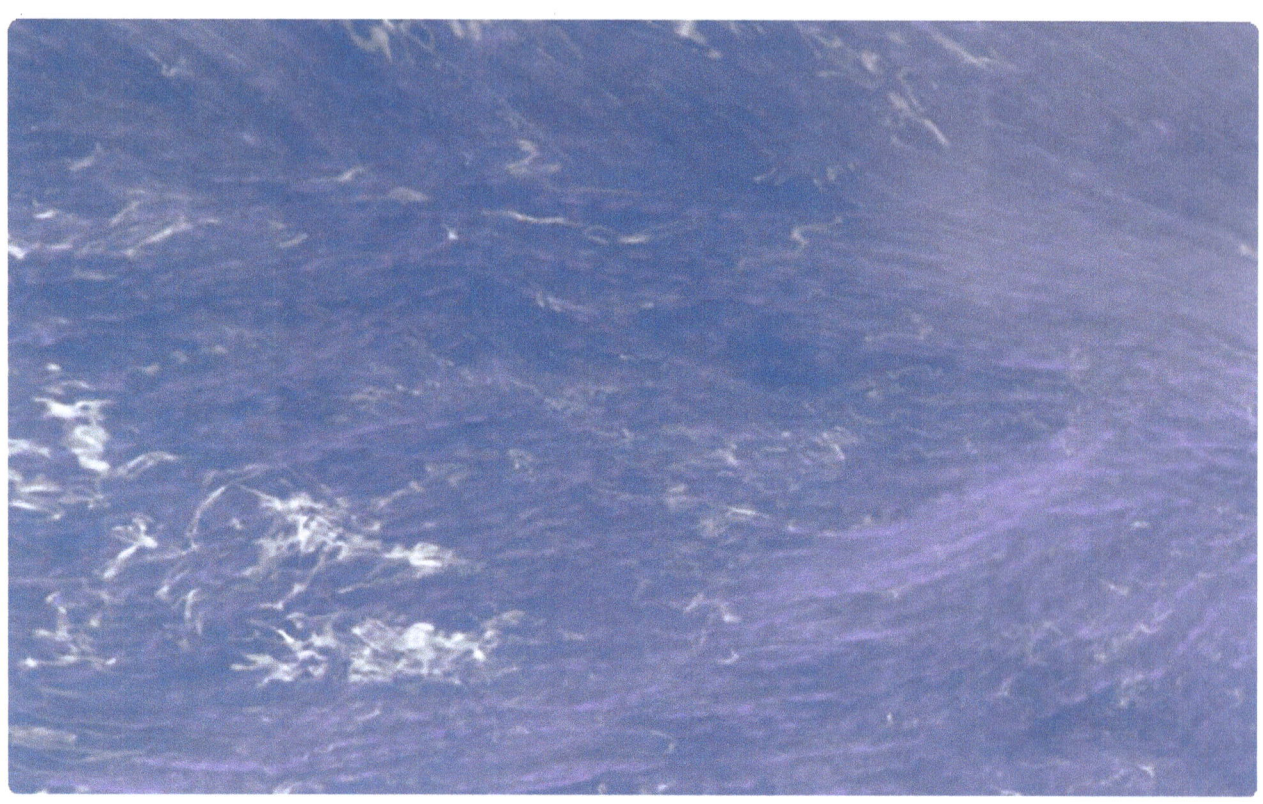

Mommy and Daddy quickly follow. After all, they see waves and deep water ahead not to mention, they always have to be on the look out for dangerous animals lurking about!

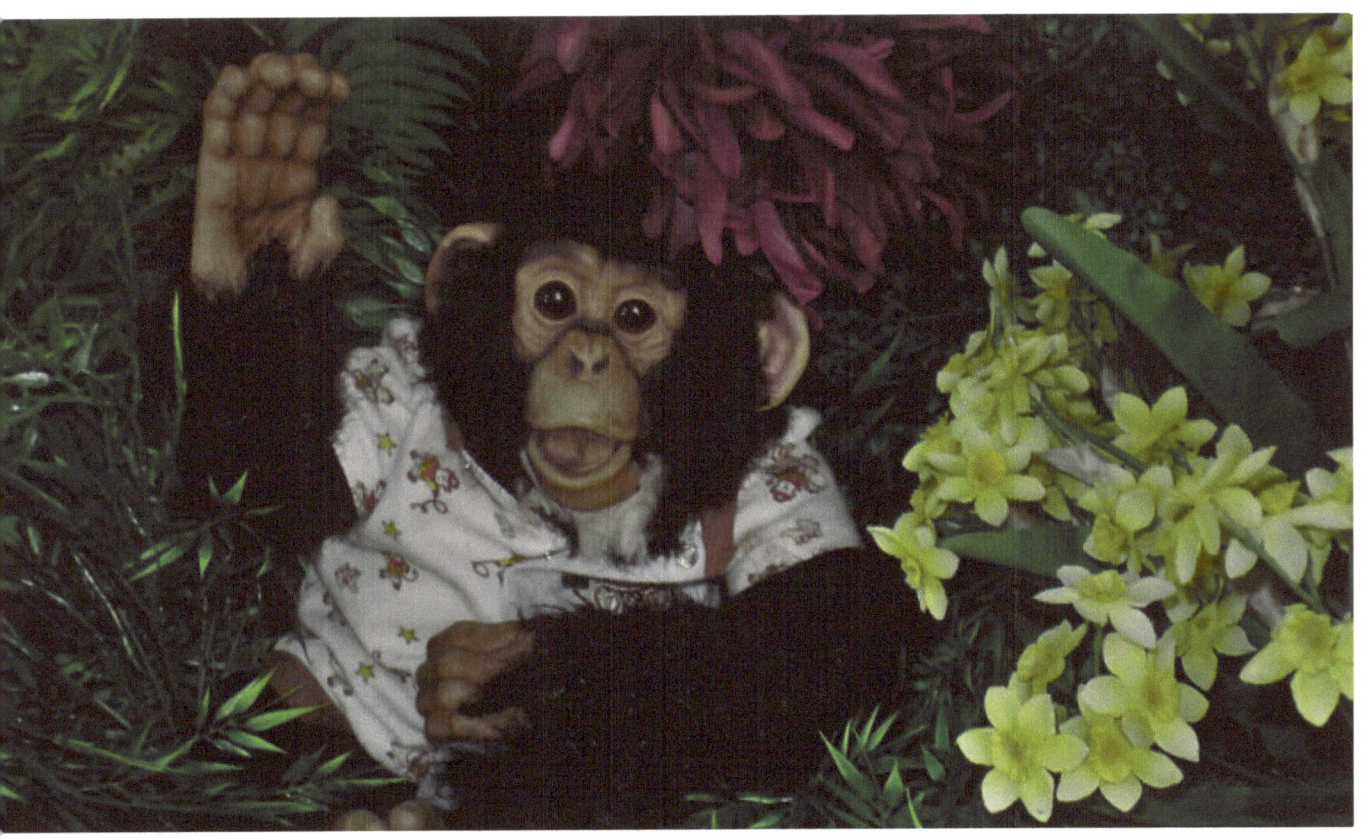

Baby Bongo is not thinking about the dangers, or the dangerous animals, he loves the waves and waves a big good bye to his parents and a little hello to his swimming instructor, Gracie, who is very serious about the rules of swimming! Like the number one rule ABC, Always Be Careful! For example, holding your breath under water too long can be dangerous! You must be careful! You can pass out when no one is looking!

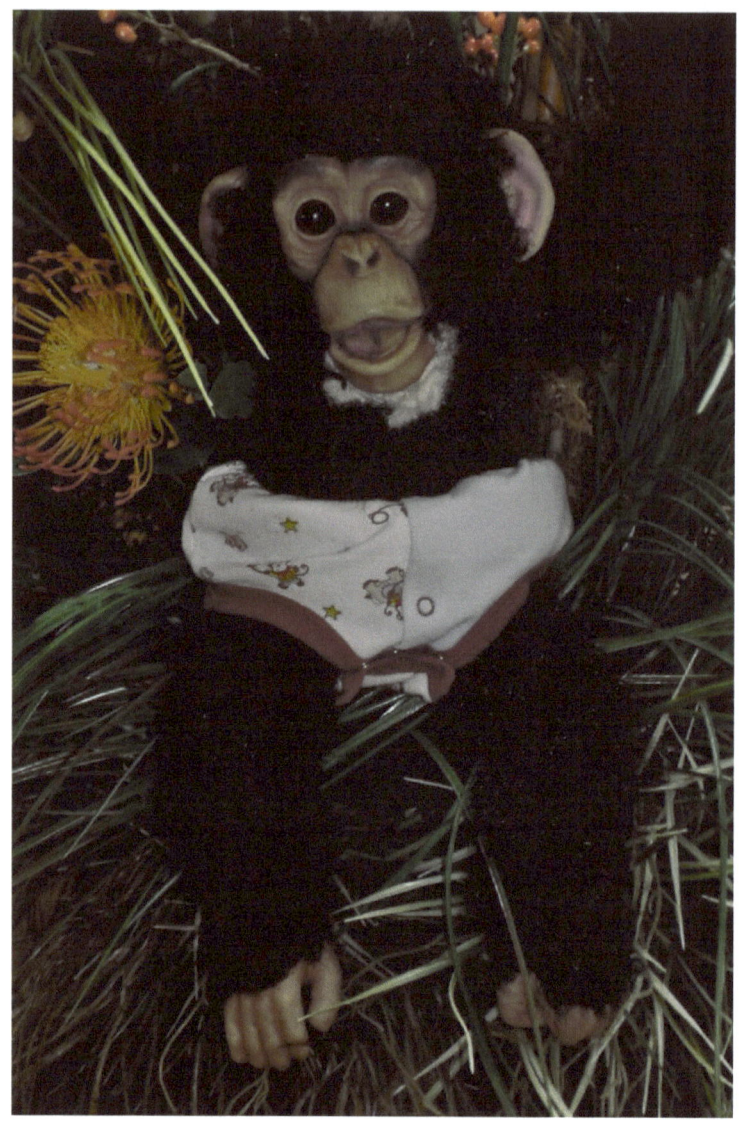

The little chimp is a bit uncooperative when it comes to listening to any rules, but Baby Bongo gets ready anyways because he is so excited to wear his new swimming shorts and learn to swim with his new teammates!

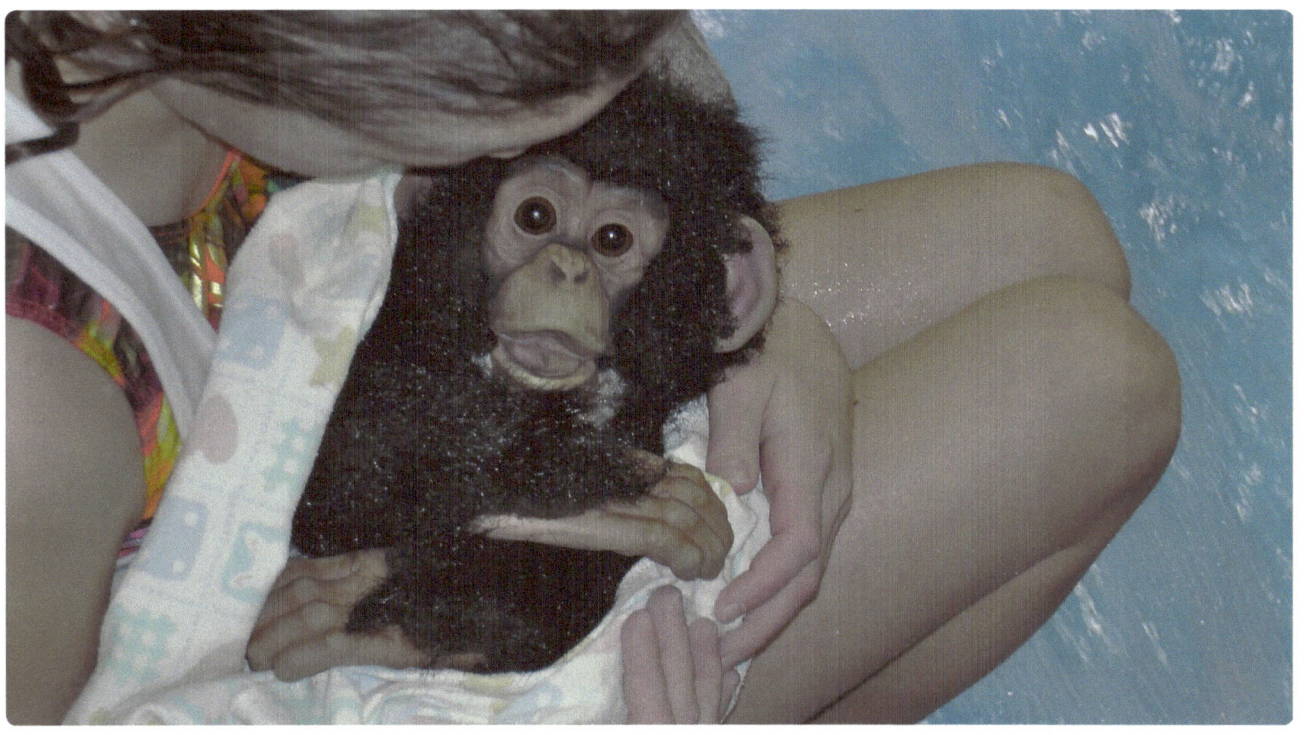

Thank goodness the little chimp loves to learn in his many lessons. Especially, with teammate Brianna, and lots of practice, he becomes a good swimmer! In fact, Baby Bongo has become such a good a swimmer, he wants to start swimming under the water right now!

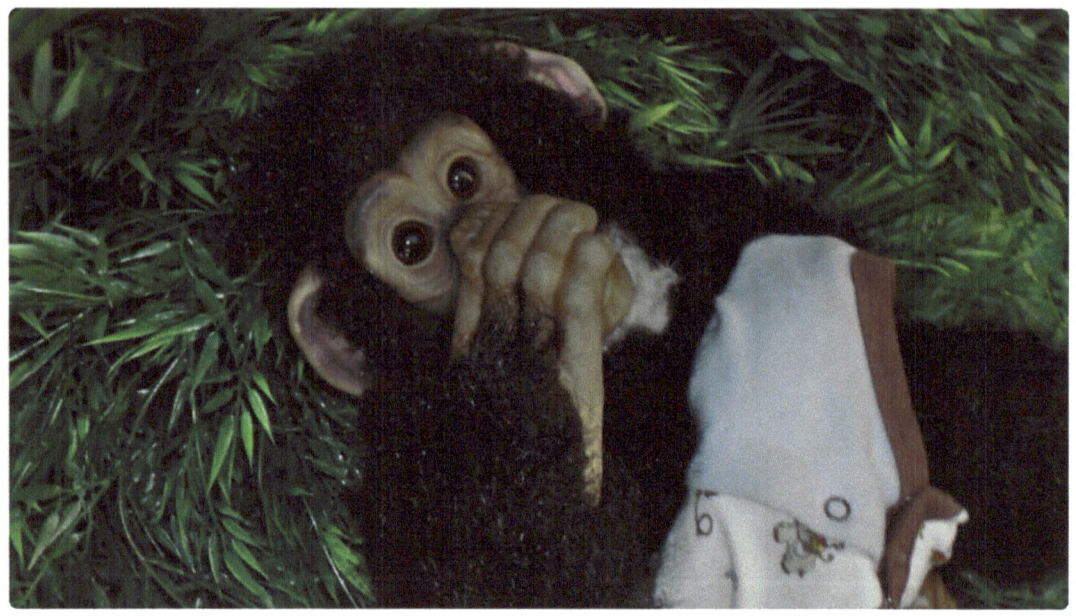

Before jumping in the water, the little chimp trades his healthy snack for an unhealthy one, with someone he barely knows! Now, instead of getting nutrition Baby Bongo gets overly excited with sugar and thinks about holding his breath the most and the longest! The little chimp remembers he could always hold his breath for a long time above water, why not under water too? Feeling mischievous, Baby Bongo looks around to make sure no one is looking at him and plans to jump in the waves and see how long he can hold his breath.

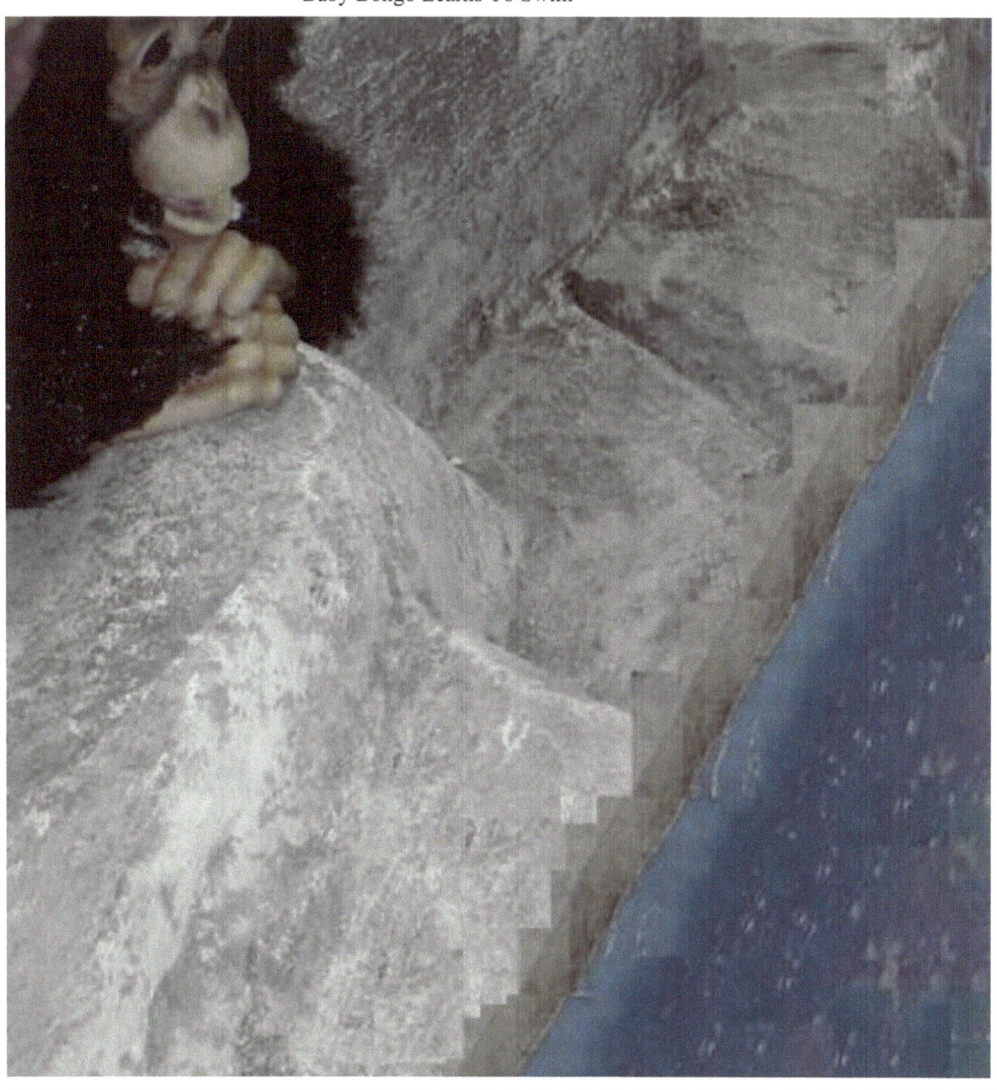

With his plan in place, Baby Bongo is more than ready, but little does the little chimp know there is an under water test in today's lessons and he is starting without instructions! Poor Baby Bongo is about to find out that holding your breath above water is very different than holding your breath under water! After all water is heavier than air and you cannot breathe the water unless you are a fish with gills!

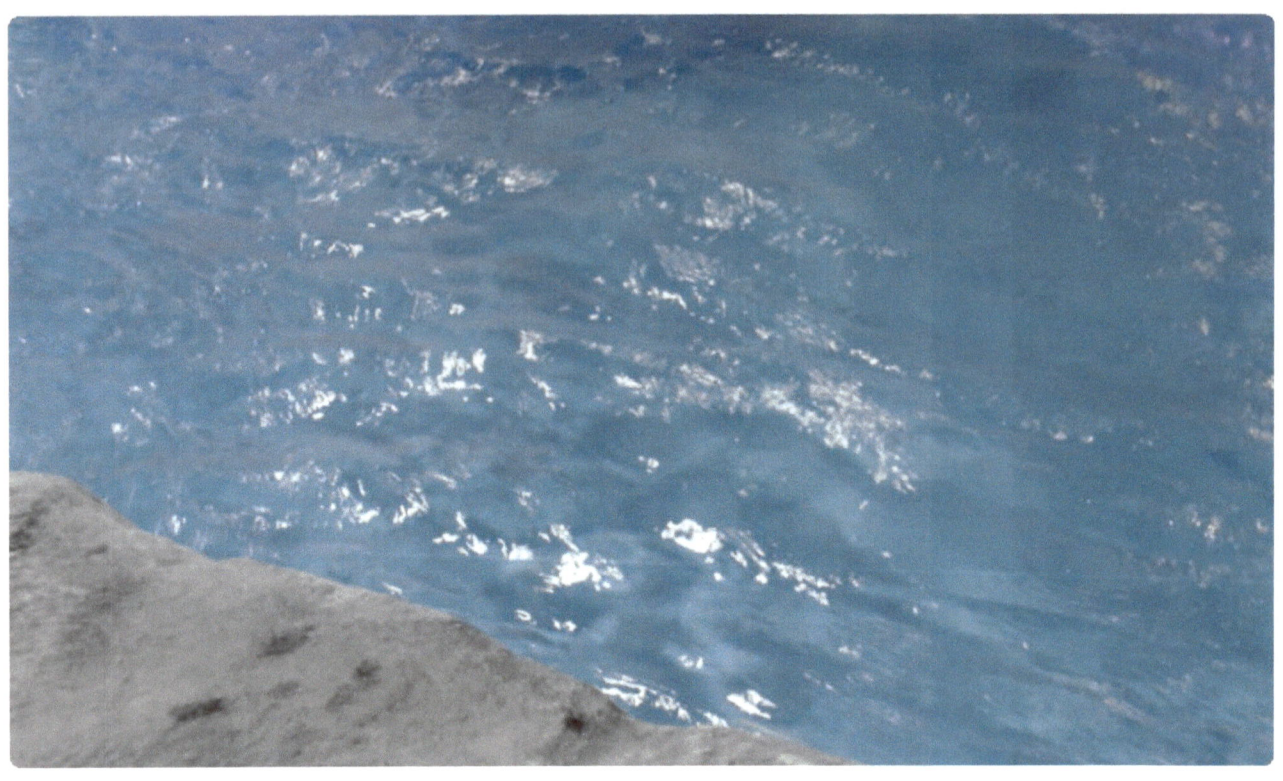

Now missing, Baby Bongo misses the instructor say, "No holding breath under water without a Buddy, it can be dangerous!". Unfortunately, Baby Bongo is already under the water holding his breath and is about to face danger!

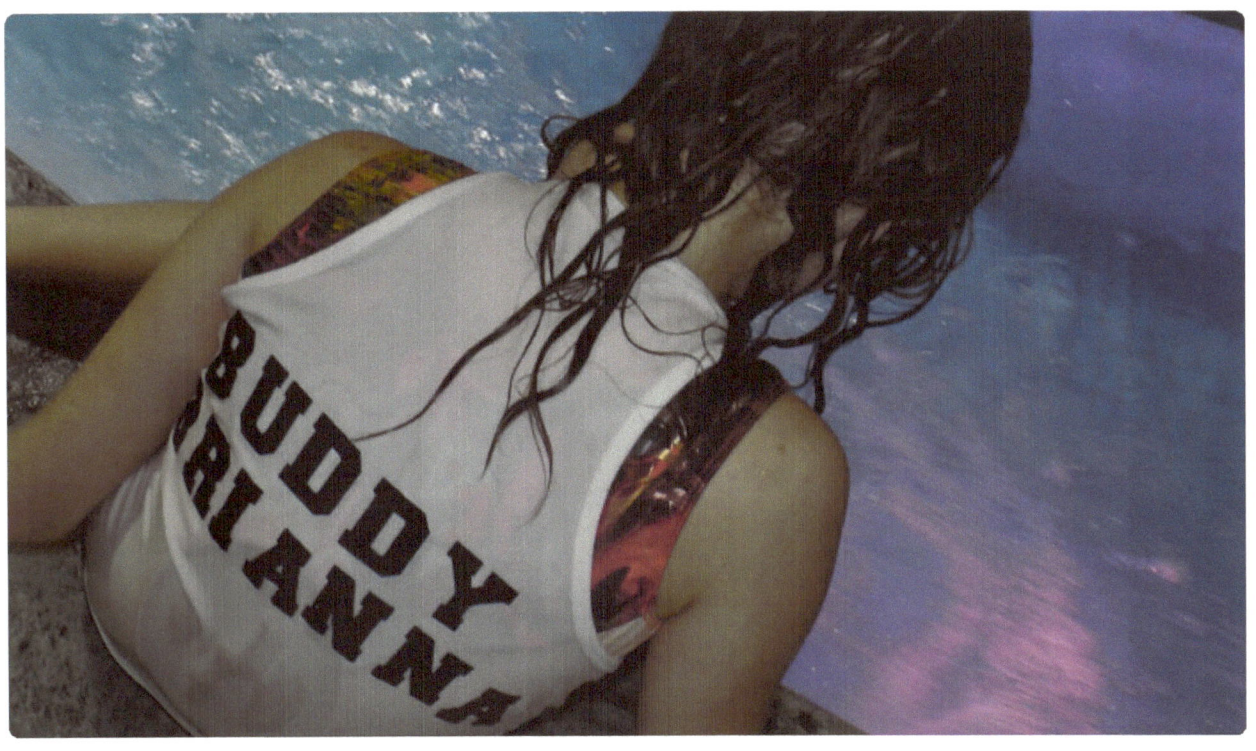

Fortunately, Baby Bongo's Buddy, who was paying attention to the instructor, hears a little splash. Then she notices Baby Bongo, under water, with his eyes closed, and not moving! The little chimp held his breath way too long. Now he was in some really deep trouble!

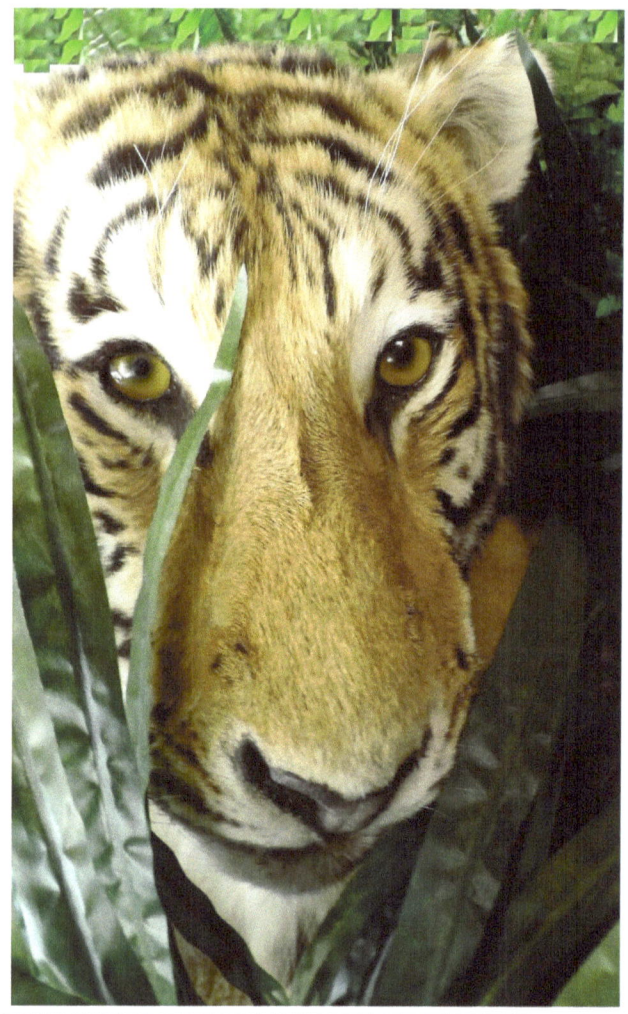

Suddenly the wind picks up and near the banks of the water there are hungry animals lurking, waiting quietly to hear any kind of splashing of their next meal. The instructor Gracie, totally serious now, also notices Baby Bongo is not moving! The instructor quickly asked Baby Bongo's Buddy, " Is the little chimp ok?", Baby Bongo's Buddy cries, "I don't think so".

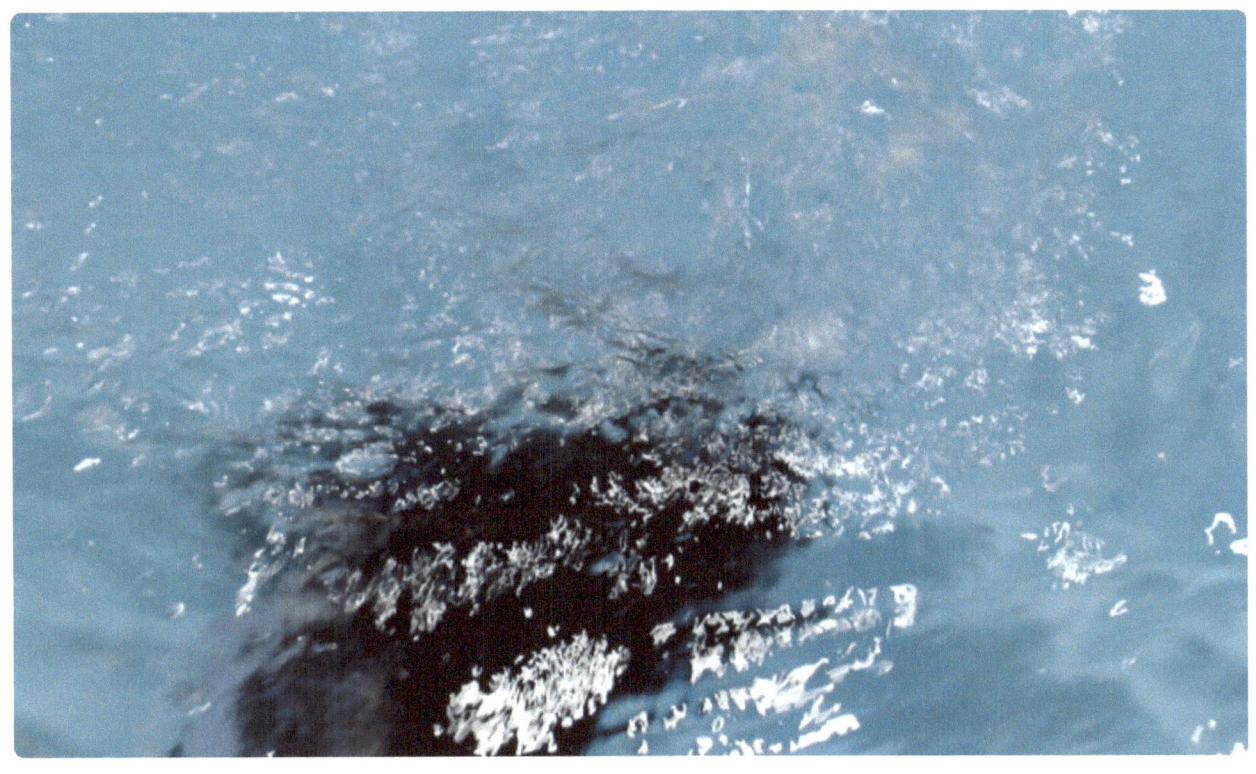

Upon hearing Baby Bongo is in trouble from his buddy Brianna, the lifeguards immediately dive in the water, acting like angels, they pull Baby Bongo out of the cold water quickly!

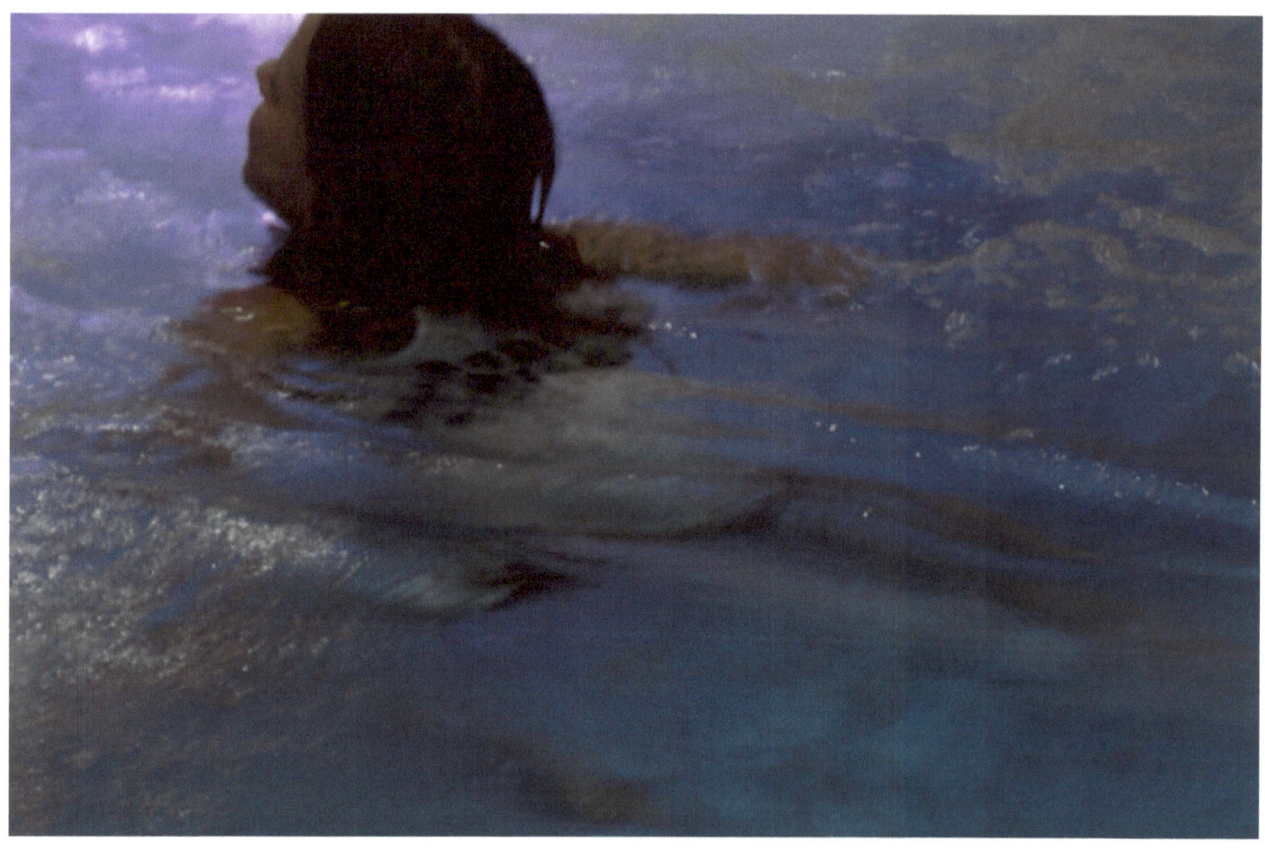

Afraid and in shock, Baby Bongo's buddy does not know what to do. She quickly climbs out of the water to find her Mommy and Daddy! After all, she just saw her buddy Baby Bongo in serious trouble and that has made her very sad!

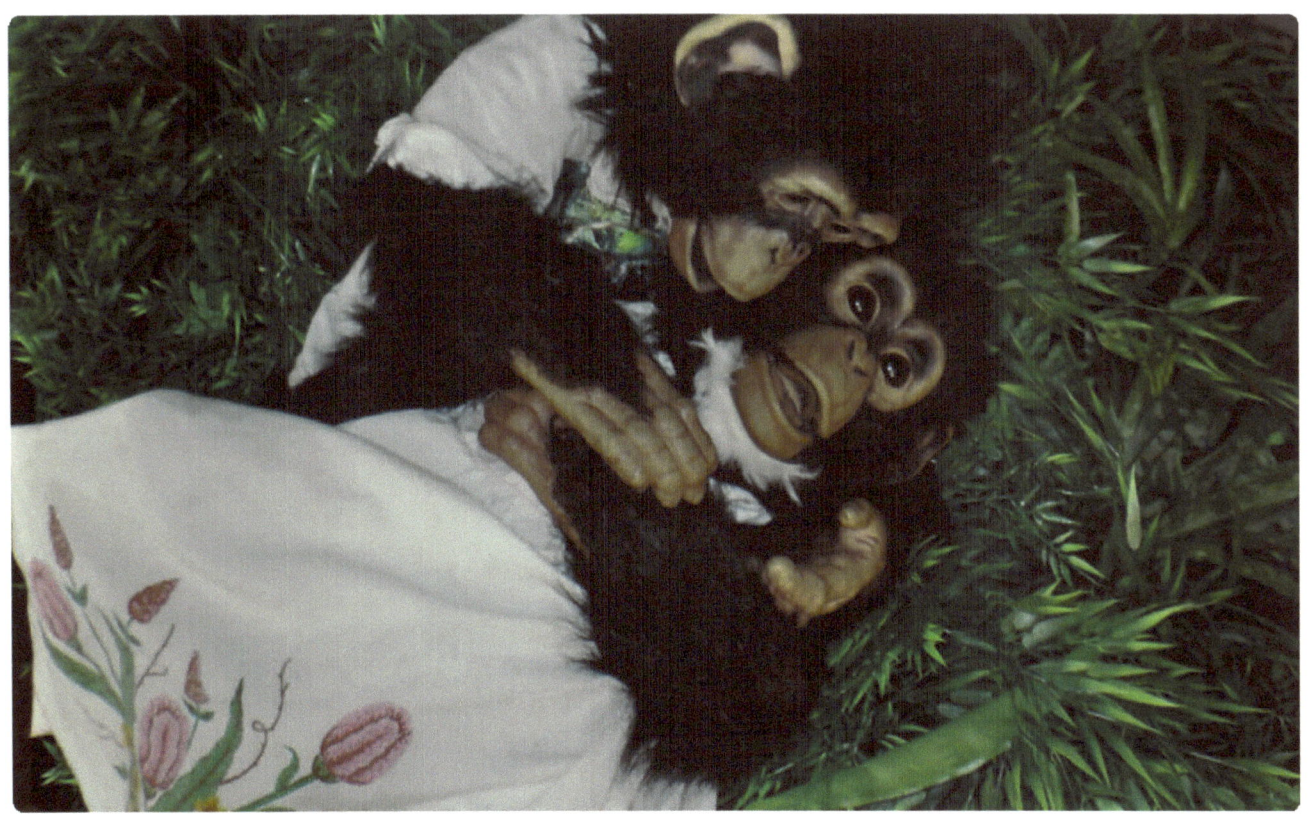

When Baby Bongo's Buddy finds her parents, she starts to cry and asks, "Did I do anything wrong?". Then she sees Baby Bongo's Mommy and Daddy looking skyward with faith and prayers, his Father is consoling his Mother, and she knows there is cause for alarm. They look very concerned, as they watch the lifeguards trying to wake Baby Bongo back up so he can breathe again!

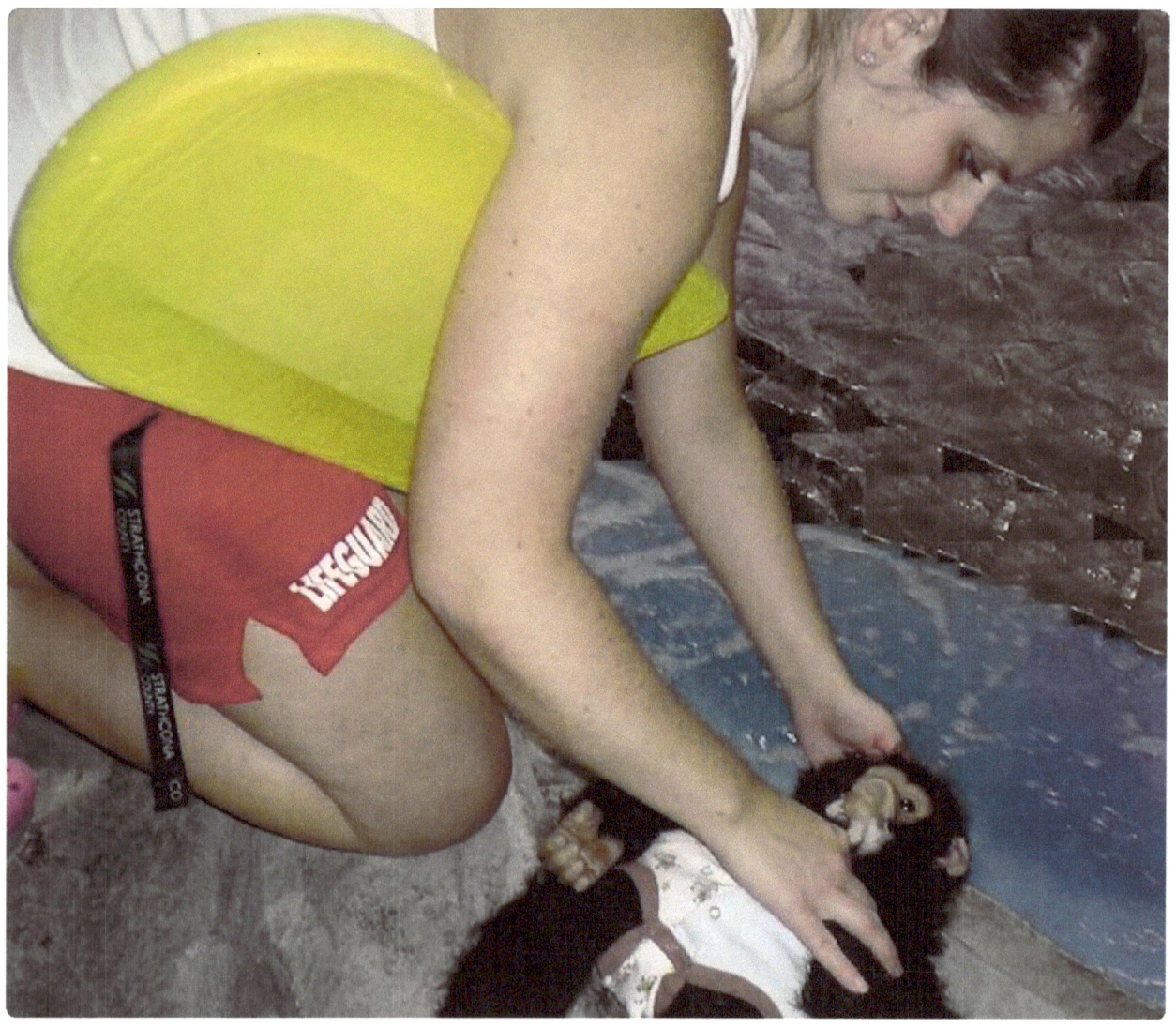

That is when Baby Bongo's Mommy saw a big sign of hope!

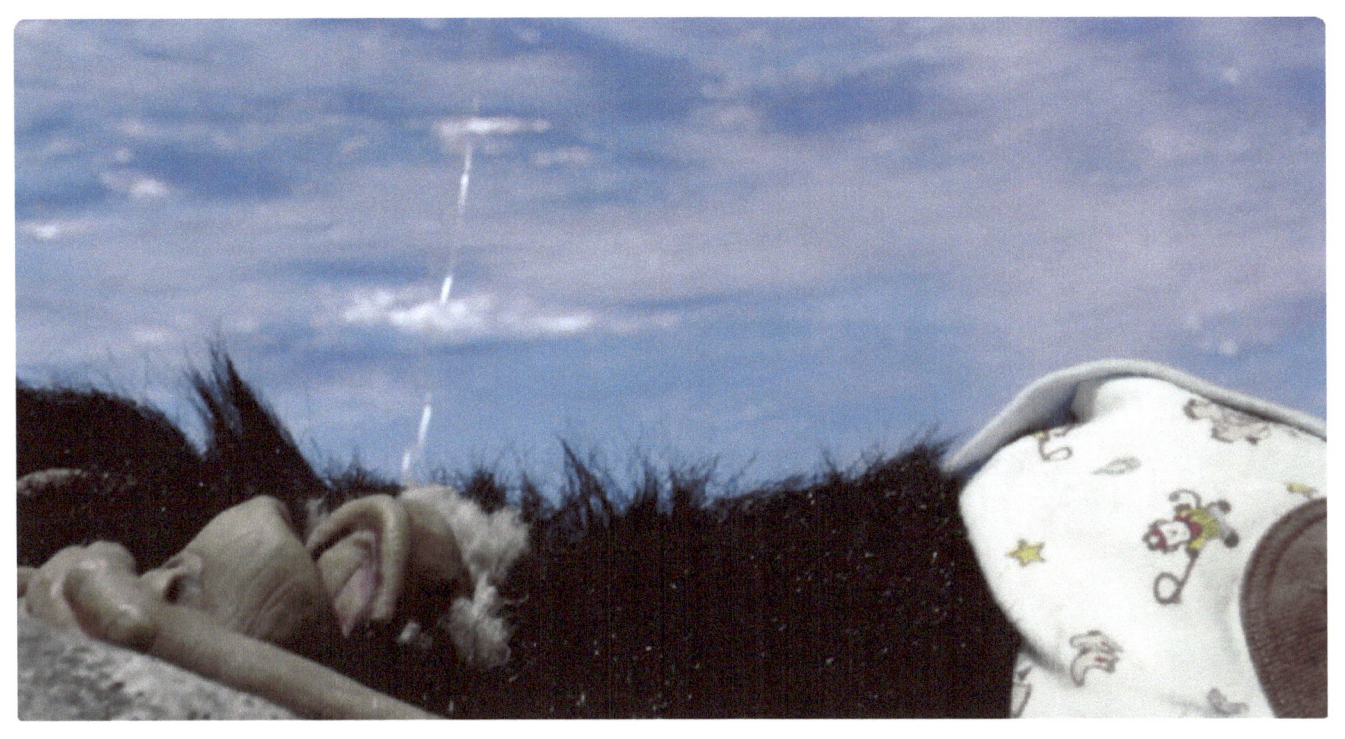

Amazingly, Baby Bongo spit water all the way to the treetops and he could breathe again! Daddy does a big flip and Mommy feels tears of joy run down her face!

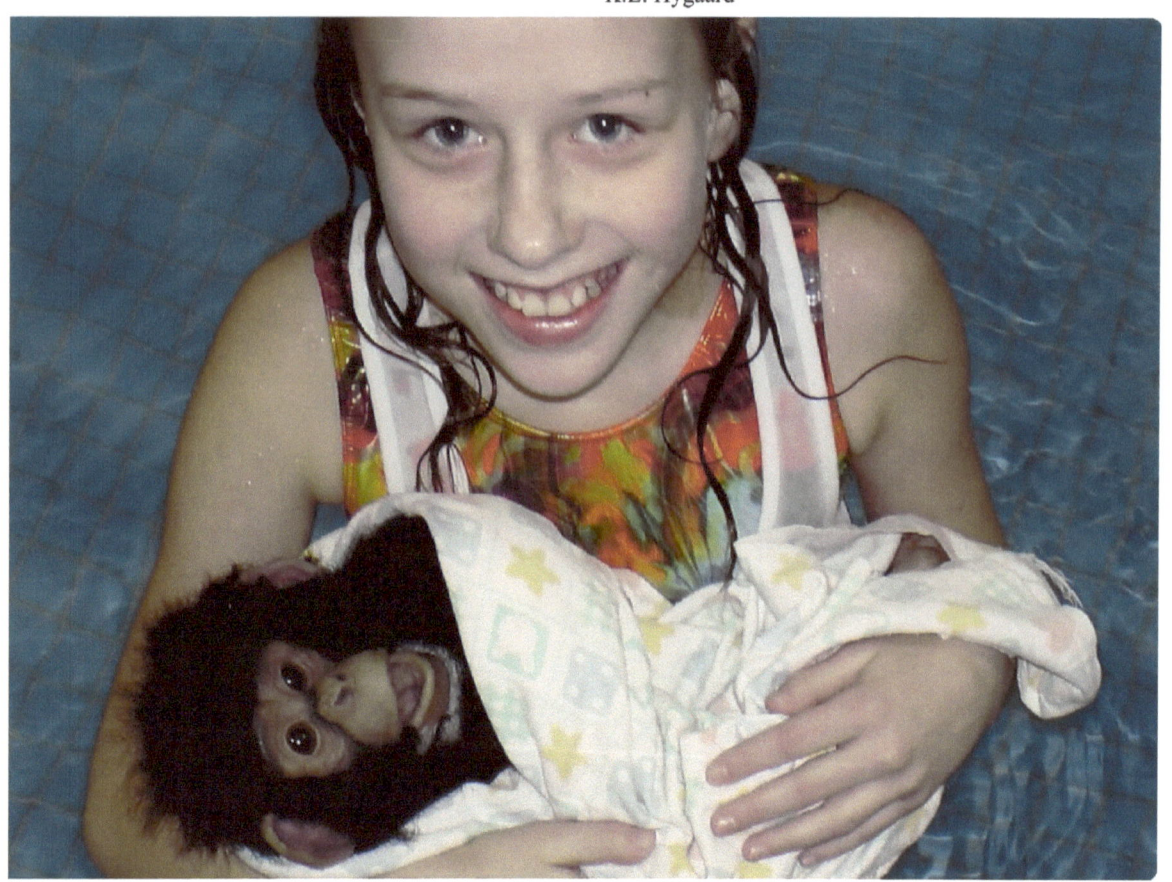

Everyone one is so happy the little chimp is okay, especially his Buddy Brianna! She finds out that she did not do anything wrong, but everything right! After all, that is what buddies do they help each other!

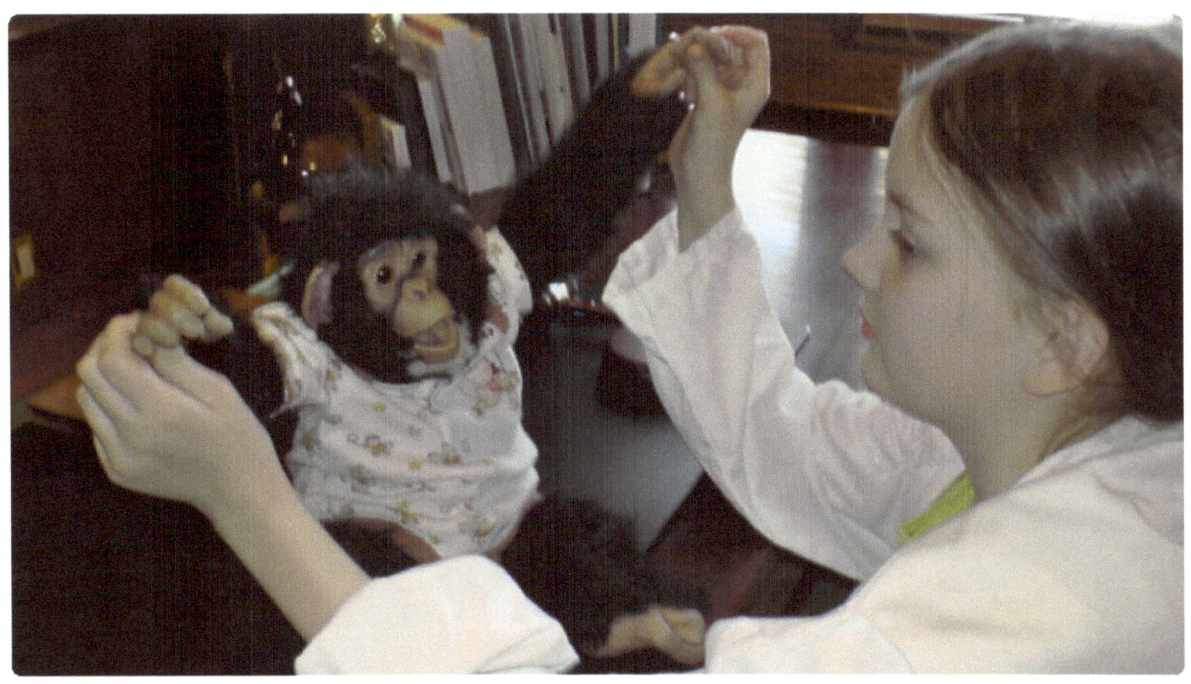

Baby Bongo's parents help too by taking their little chimp to visit Dr. V. Vet! Mommy and Daddy want to make sure Baby Bongo is okay before bedtime! After the doctor was able to help the little chimp get the rest of the water out of his lungs, she recommended the little chimp get back on the healthy path, as soon as possible!

Baby Bongo learned that when you are involved in any sport and you want to be the best you can be, eating right and having proper rest is the key to success! Not to mention how rules can save lives!

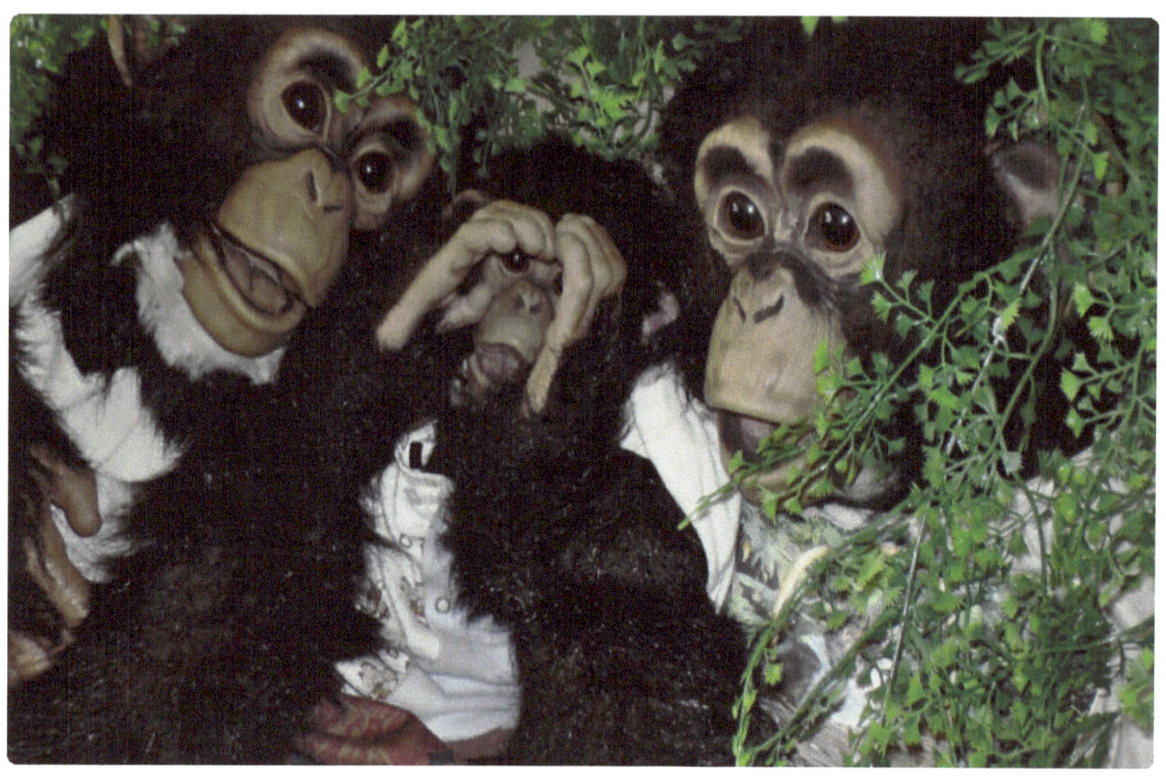

The next morning, after a peaceful sleep and healthy breakfast, Baby Bongo's parents told him about the many things that happened while he was recovering. They told the little chimp that, because of his accident there would no longer be underwater testing at swimming lessons. "Why?" Baby Bongo asked. After all, Baby Bongo did not really remember what happened."Because, Baby Bongo, we love you and do not want bad things to happen to you".

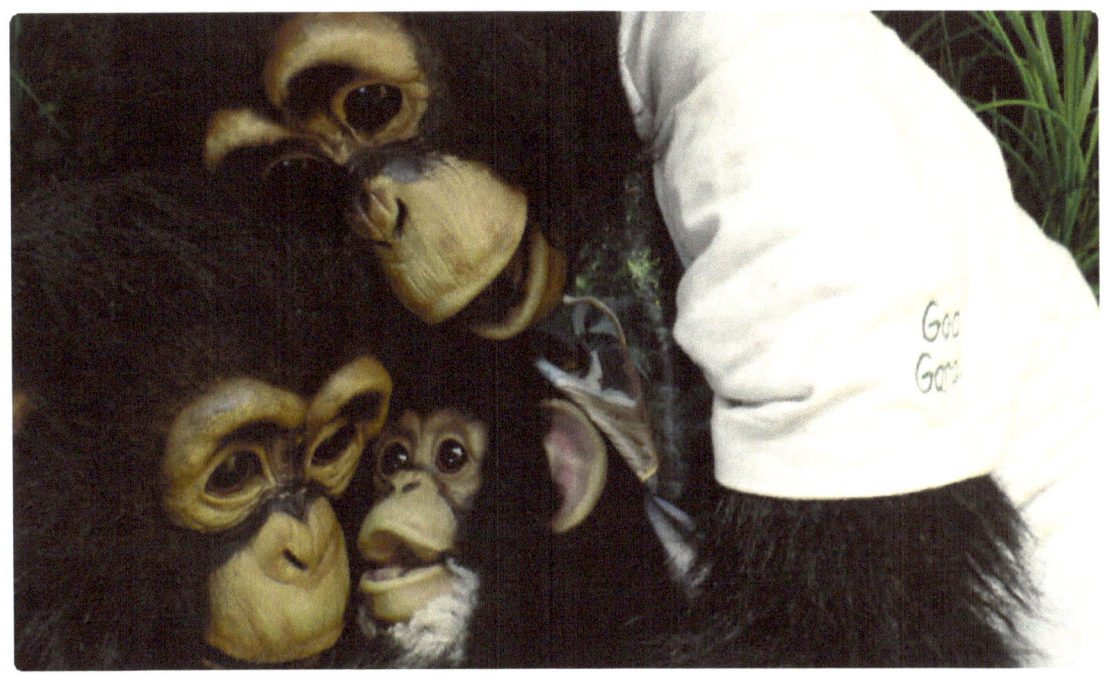

"I love you too, Mommy and Daddy", says Baby Bongo, as he hugs tight! Snug and warm, Marimba and Viola give thanks to all those who watched over their little Baby Bongo when they could not. "I saw a Giraffe under water!" Baby Bongo whispers to his Mommy, "and then I saw a big hand reaching down for me!" Marimba and Viola smile and remind Baby Bongo he is loved and to stay on the healthy path, it will make his life much better!

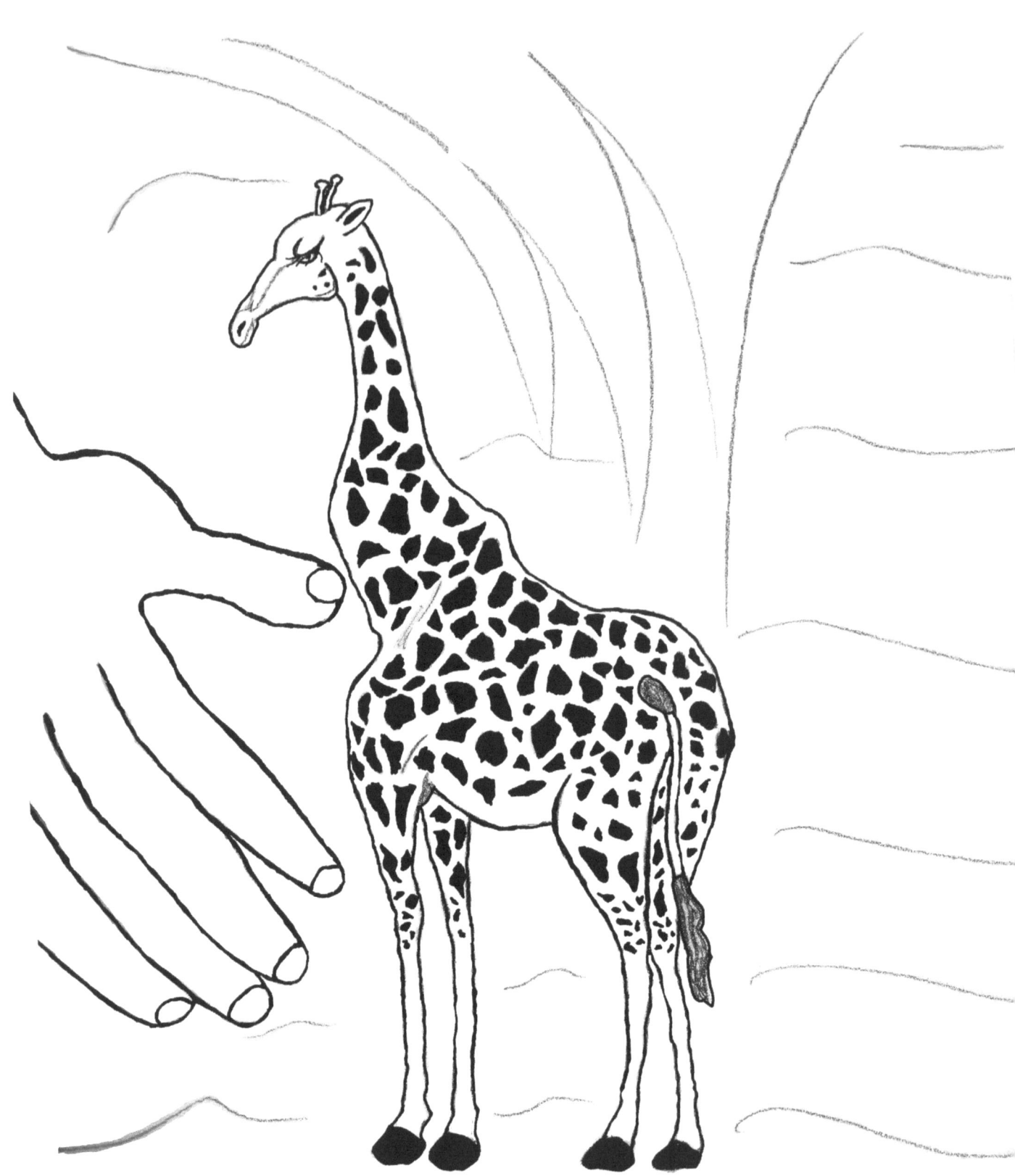

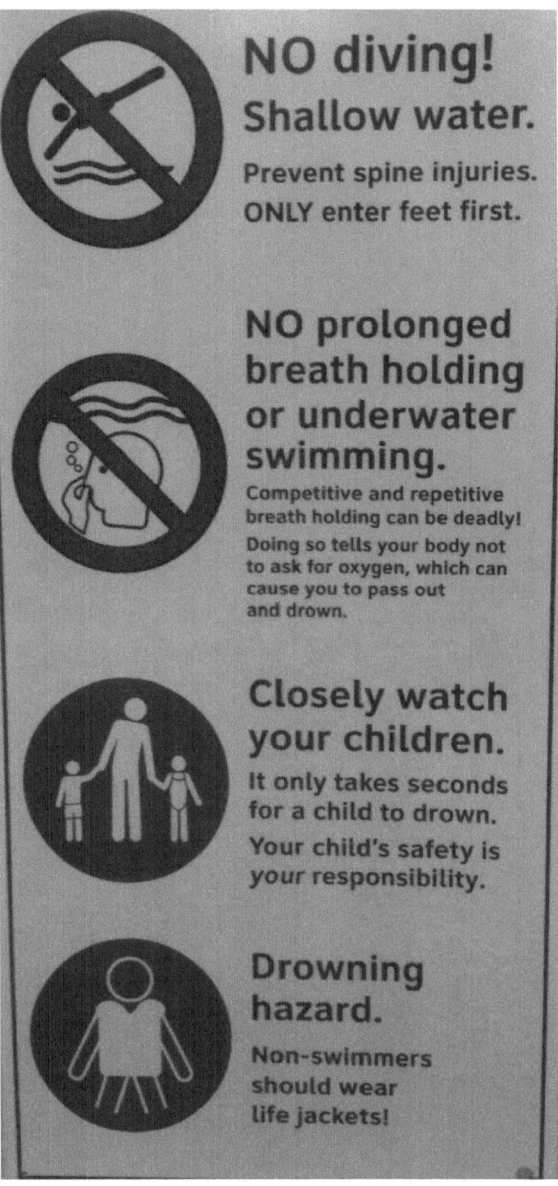

On the Healthy Path you feel better about following Rules

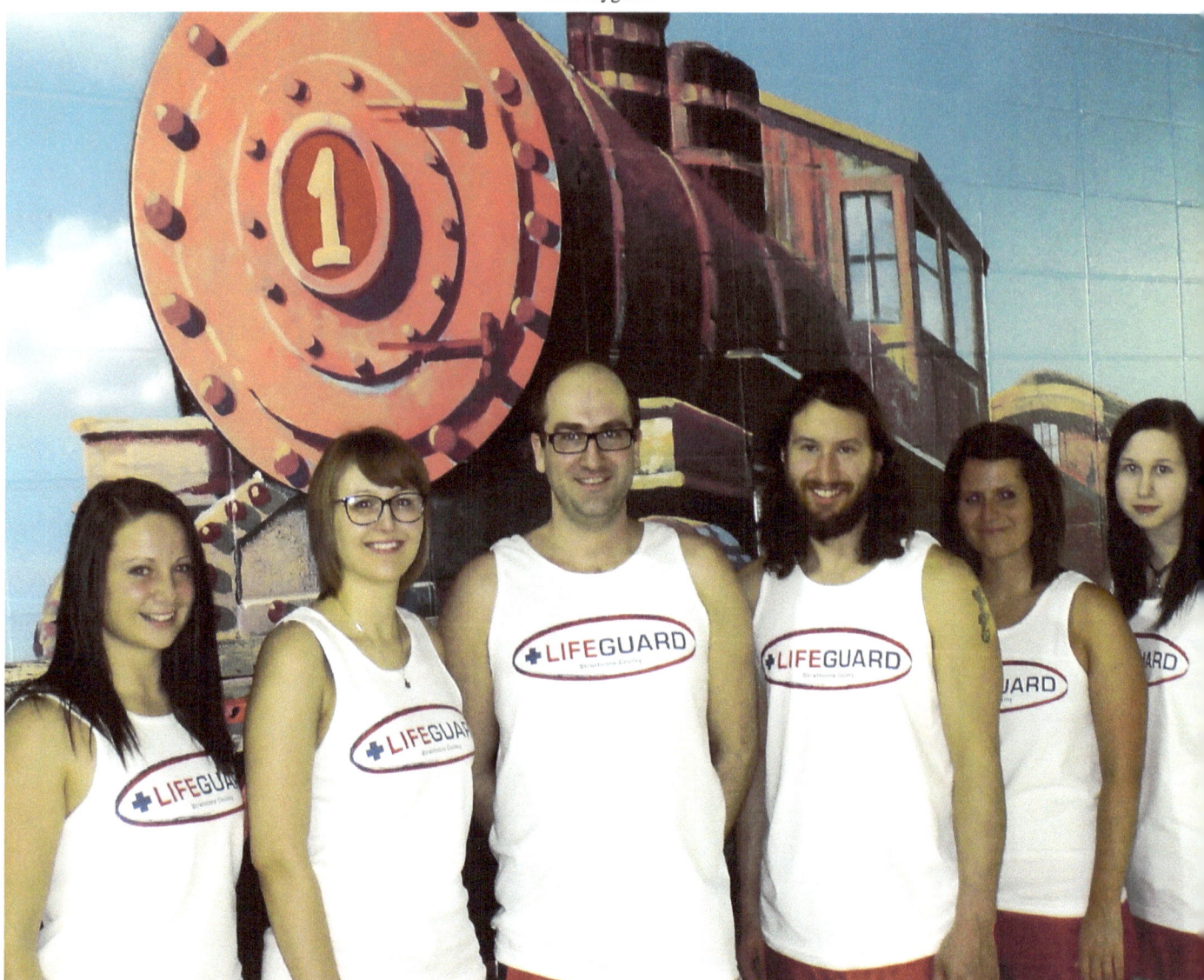

A heartfelt Thank You to the Lifeguards on Duty and whose efforts changed our lives by rescuing Ruscita!

DEDICATION

I would like to dedicate this book to my daughter for her courage to get back in the water and Brianna for looking out for others! You never know when you maybe saving a life!

Acknowledgements

A Sincere Thank you to Family & Friends for all their Support and Prayers! Faith brings Peace of Mind!

Special Thanks

I would also like to thank all those who acted quickly to save my daughter's life! From the lifeguards to the first responders taking her in the ambulance to the nice medical staff at the University of Alberta hospital and her supportive club members.

ABOUT THE AUTHOR

K.L. Hygaard was born in Edmonton, Alberta, Canada. Being a Canadian she has spent some time in New Brunswick and Newfoundland traveling through the wilderness developing ideas for her art, with continued trips home to Alberta to spend time with family and the wilds of the surrounding region. Recently she traveled to Quebec City for three years where she discovered a place flourishing with ideas and unique cultural influences. She has been entertaining with puppets since the age of three and her first show was at age six, she has continued performing ever since. She studied acting in Vancouver and Los Angeles in order to grow as an artist and she continues working live shows to deliver the messages of health and wellness. While living and working in Nashville as a children's entertainer, K. L. Hygaard created the idea for Brigitta's Mystical Garden. Currently she lives in Edmonton working on the series. Website: *www.bmgchild.com*